Table Of Contents

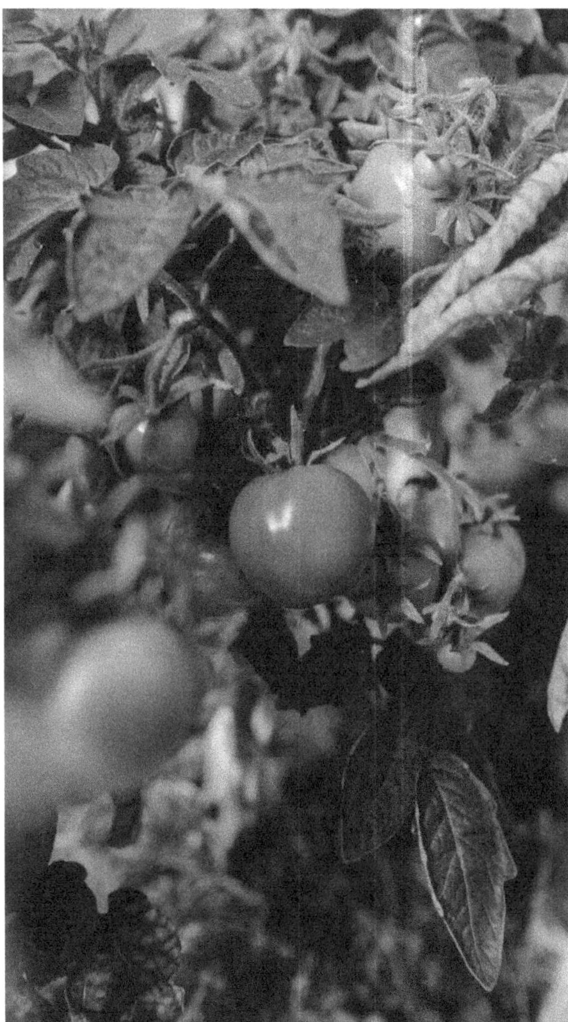

Foreword

This may be the most important and simple-to-understand information you'll ever read on battling or preventing cancer. You can take effective action to beat cancer after you are aware of the underlying causes of the disease and what you can do to address those causes.

Finding out you or a loved one has cancer can be a terrifying experience. However, if you understand what causes cancer,

You or a loved one may have a better than average chance of beating cancer if you identify the causes of the disease and figure out how to stop them.

Unfortunately, not everyone can survive using these methods, but if the individual

Utilizing these techniques has enough time to start working, they frequently reverse their cancer.

You can safely increase the likelihood of avoiding cancer even if you're undergoing routine medical procedures or simply attempting to avoid getting it.

Utilizing some of the ideas discussed here will increase the effectiveness of what you accomplish.

How To Treat Cancer Without Drugs.

The Best Advice For Avoiding This Killer

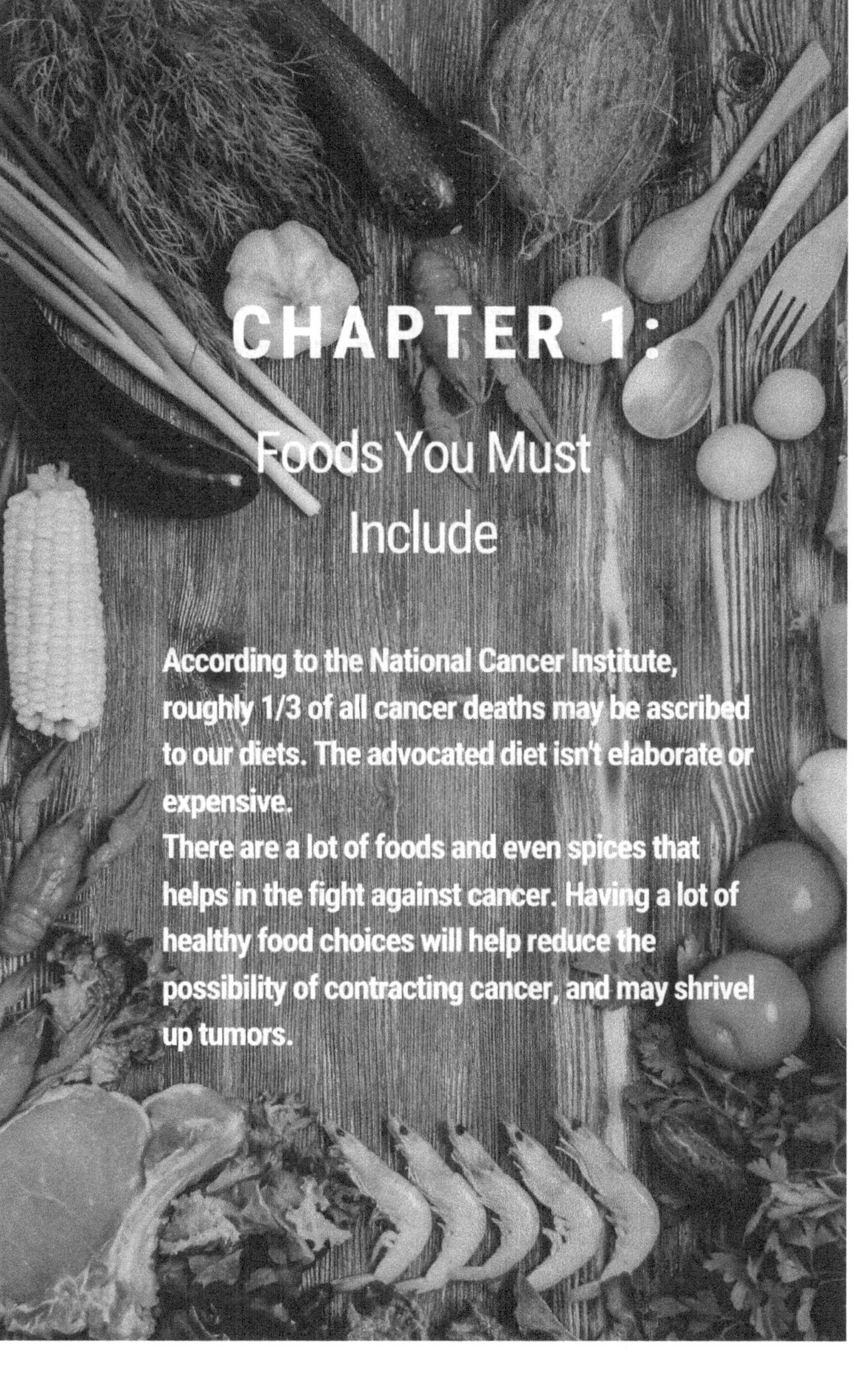

CHAPTER 1:
Foods You Must Include
According to the National Cancer Institute, roughly 1/3 of all cancer deaths may be ascribed to our diets. The advocated diet isn't elaborate or expensive.
There are a lot of foods and even spices that helps in the fight against cancer. Having a lot of healthy food choices will help reduce the possibility of contracting cancer, and may shrivel up tumors.

Eat Right

Numerous factors affect the development of cancer. The Mayo Clinic postulates that unhealthy diet, obesity, and smoking promote cancer. Additionally, for some types of cancer, genetic endowment plays a role. It's easy enough to safeguard yourself against skin cancer. In order to shield your skin from UV rays during the day, you need to wear sunscreen.

Brussel sprouts, kale, broccoli, and other cruciferous vegetables both include two important antioxidants: lutein and zeaxanthin. Prostate cancer may be fought off with the aid of these antioxidants. Several of the market's fresh vegetables are loaded with vitamins, antioxidants, and minerals, which could help in cancer prevention.

The immune system is boosted by oranges and lemons to fight cancer cells. Ascorbic acid, an antioxidant, is present in papayas. Raspberries are rich in vitamins and minerals that help keep the body healthy against cancer. The abundance of antioxidants in nuts may help to reduce the expansion of tumors.

According to scientific research, tea has the ability to combat cancer. Green tea is produced from unfermented tea leaves, yet all teas are beneficial to health. As a result, it has the highest antioxidant density. Polyphenols are the name for the antioxidants found in tea.

An article published by the University of Maryland Medical Center in 2007 According to the Center, polyphenols are known to fight free radicals.Free radicals are produced naturally by the body, but many diseases, including cancer, are thought to be caused primarily by them.

Green tea's polyphenols may balance these free radicals, and could potentially lessen or stop physical harm from occurring.

Some scientific researchers claim that allum chemicals found in garlic appear to aid the immunological system. Turmeric, which belongs to the ginger family, also aids in the fight against cancer. spiciest chile chiles and Capsaicin, which is found in jalapenos and is known to be a cancer preventative agent. Rosemary, a fragrant spice, could be useful in the fight against cancer

CHAPTER 2:

Skip Breakfast

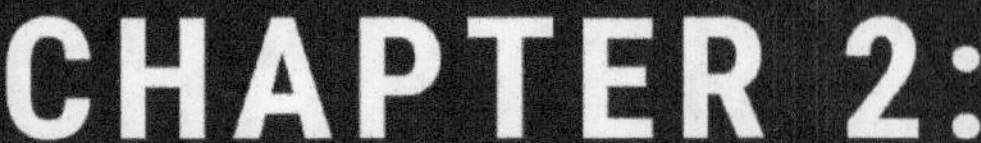

Fasting is the panacea for preventing and reversing all sorts of metabolic dysfunction and health issues.

Be willing to change or you perish.

Fast

Is breakfast the most important meal of the day?
I think every meal you eat is important

Let me explain

You are only in control of your food, when it has not left your plate to your mouth. The moment it leaves your plate to your mouth you seized to be in control enzymes, hormones and other internal processes beyond your control happens.

The concept of breakfast didn't exist until around the industrial age. Where fast life and convenience became a norm. Let me chip in a little physiology here It will take between 20-30 hours for food to move from your mouth to your Anus. First 3-12hours between your stomach and your colon. The remaining hours in your colon. You need a space between each meal. At least for your stomach and intestine to work effectively.

Modern advice is that you should eat breakfast between 7 am and 9 am. Not bad advice though.

Now here is where the problem lies, in most mornings you won't have time to cook good food, that gives you a fast alternative

-Bread
-Breakfast cereals
-noodles

All high carbs high fat

Your body has enough calories in store to take you up to 10days without harm, your blood can only hold 4g of glucose in a given time. That's 1 cube of sugar, your liver stores up to 100g of glycogen(liver starch). Your muscles stores a further 300g of glucose. When you eat every time you don't allow your body to utilize fat, because glucose is always present in your blood, which the body responds by producing insulin, insulin helps your body utilize nutrients, insulin promotes fat storage(anabolism), the fat you are not using.

Overtime eating leads to more production of insulin, your cells start getting tired of insulin and resist it.

Leading to your pancreas, producing more,half of your problem will be solved if you cut out sugar, further 20% if you delay the next meal, 25% percent if you sourced your calories from

-Protein
-non Starchy veggies
-good fats

If you eat

-Fibre
-organic foods

Breakfast 1: 11-12 am

Breakfast 2: before 8 pm

Make sure at least 2 hours before bedtime.

"Can I add muscle when I fast?"

I get this question all the time.

The answer is YES.

"Will I not become thin if I fast?"

The answer is NO.

Fasting does not make you thin.

Fasting cleans your gut and makes your metabolic machinery efficient. When you start fasting, you will lose weight. This weight is called 'water weight'.

Water weight is water that has been pooled by the glycogen in your body because glycogen is hydrophilic (It loves water), the body will lose weight up to its lowest threshold and then begins bulking up.

More reasons why you should take fasting serious..

- Fasting will optimize your Testosterone.

- Fasting will improve your metabolism.

- Fasting will improve your sleep.

- Fasting will improve your gut health.

- Fasting will improve your cognitive functions.

-Fasting will improve your immunity.

-Fasting will improve your emotional IQ.

- Fasting will improve your spirituality.

- Fasting will reduce unnecessar cravings

-Fasting will improve your HDL

No hospital will tell you this.

Decide to make shrewd changes today.

CHAPTER 3:

Chemicals Are Not Your Friend.

Every day, contaminants and toxins are introduced into our homes through water, food, dirt, dust, and household cleaning supplies.
For instance, several antiseptics, air fresheners, and disinfectants may include the dangerous toxin phenol. Continuing to be exposed to phenols and further

Toxins could harm our nervous and respiratory systems as well as cause cancer. To reduce your danger and exposure, it's critical to educate oneself.

You might wish to replace some of the harmful agents you find with non-toxic alternatives after you start to educate yourself on the chemicals and toxins listed on the labels of the products in your home.

No Toxins

To be sure you're not using home products that contain harmful pollutants, carefully examine the list of ingredients on all of their labels. You should keep this website in your folder, to search for products that meet the safer choice standard to check how safe your home products are
https://www.epa.gov/saferchoice/products

Choose your seafood wisely to reduce the amount of mercury you absorb. Limit your consumption of canned tuna, stay away from shark, swordfish, and bluefish, and opt instead for wild salmon, tilapia, or Pacific cod. Use grilling, broiling, or roasting cooking methods instead of frying meals. When choosing fruits and vegetables that would ordinarily have the greatest pesticide levels, try to buy organic if at all possible.

Install a water filter to shield you from heavy metals. Searching for "water filter comparisons" on Google will yield a large number of websites from which to choose, all of which will allow you to compare the performance ratings of many leading brands of water filters.
Make an effort to use Teflon or any other non-stick pans as little as possible.

According to the Environmental Working Group, this cookware more quickly achieves temperatures that produce harmful gasses and particulates. For your cookware, you might wish to choose cast iron or stainless steel.

Never put plastic in the microwave. Use "microwave safe" packaging or glass or ceramic containers, as appropriate. Although the literature is debatable, several health advocacy groups believe that microwave cooking releases dioxin into plastic.

Be cautious while using antibacterial soaps. They might include environmentally harmful pesticides that can be absorbed through the skin. Use a straightforward soap and water to scrub your hands for 20 seconds.

Make an effort to use fewer pesticides and herbicides. Both skin contact and inhalation are ways that harmful substances might enter our bodies. Before entering the home, take off your shoes. Pesticides from lawns, invisible chemicals on the ground, and outdoor dust can all be readily brought back into your home and last there for a very long time.

Limit your use of bleach and instead use lemon juice to whiten teeth. Don't believe the advertising just because a select few businesses are benefiting from excellent "green marketing tricks." Read the instructions on all of your detergent's bottles. Avoid adding any softeners to your washer or dryer to reduce the number of chemicals that come into contact with your garments. To prevent some of the chemicals and odors from reentering your home, leave any clothes that have been professionally washed outside for around eight hours.

Always vacuum with a filter in it, preferably a HEPA filter. Small particles that ordinary vacuums might pump back into your home's air are captured by a HEPA filter. You should regularly vacuum and dust your home because there may be a variety of allergies present, including dust mites.
Choose personal care and cosmetics made by businesses that don't use hazardous ingredients. You can study information about items you are considering buying or that you are currently using on the web to check for known or suspected risks. Despite a product's low danger designation on a website, there is no assurance that it is secure. The products indicated in the low hazard groups should also be checked for safety.

CHAPTER 4:

Put Down The Smokes

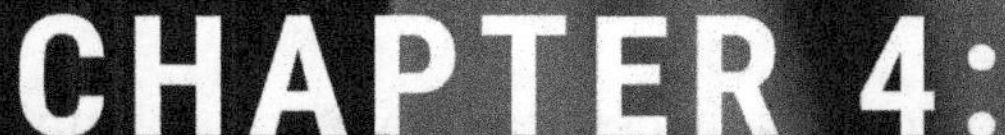

No more chesty coughs. Stop giving money to "XYZ
Tobacco" on a daily basis. Breathing difficulties and
social isolation are no longer an issue.
It's time to give up smoking permanently.
 Down The Smokes

Quit

The most important piece of advice I can give you is what I like to call the "Why."

Ask yourself, "What motivated me to quit smoking?"

Now, in order to be more fit and to create a better environment or to save money, to have healthy children, the list goes on. When your Why isn't firm, you won't adhere to it. Say, for instance, that you established a goal but never followed through on it? For sure I know I have, as do most people.

Why do we sometimes follow through on our goals while doing so other times? It is as a result of the underlying reason. If quitting smoking is motivated by your confidence and honestly believing you're powerful, you're a lot more likely to be an abstainer.

Put your why down and keep it nearby where you keep your cigarettes. One example may be, "I'm going to stop smoking because of........."

Your causes have a lot of force! Different people stop for a variety of reasons. So it's important to include your own motivations in your essay. When assessing your arguments, be careful that they are not motivated by pressure from friends, family, or coworkers because this will make it harder for you to stick to your position. You must choose to stop smoking on your own terms, not solely on the opinions of others.

If you carry cigarettes simply because they are available. In order to ensure that you don't allow it to influence you, it's essential to throw away your smokes and lighter. Put your usual cigarette spending cash in a jar. This is an extremely effective tactic because many smokers don't sit down and calculate how much they actually spend on smokes each year. You're more likely to stay motivated if you can practically see the money you'd have spent on cigarettes. It's highly effective once you let people know that you've already given up.

It has less impact when people say, "I'm attempting to stop smoking." When someone claims they're attempting to halt something, it offers them the justification for saying, "Well, it didn't work, but I tried!" Even though we don't always realize it, we are proud of ourselves when man achieves goals. In light of this, once you admit quitting, If your Why is to smoke, make sure you're proud of it and reward yourself with the money you've set aside.

You might have developed the attitude of light up when you wake up, get in the car, sip coffee, after a meal, or when you're under stress. Replace the cigarette when you wake up in the morning with a glass of water. When the itches appear or urge to smoke, change your behavior in any way that keeps you from smoking.

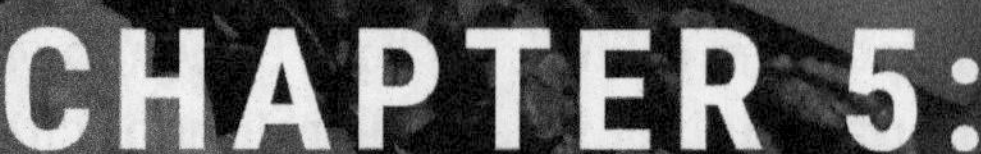

CHAPTER 5:

Fibre Is Your Friend

Recent studies support what nutritionists have been saying for years: eating a lot of high-fiber meals is a great strategy to safeguard your health. That assertion might seem bold. But it's the facts, said researchers leading the largest-ever investigation into the link between nutrition and cancer.

Use Fiber

Some people might believe that fiber's ability to fight cancer is still up for debate. However, given the numerous benefits of foods high in fiber, such as whole grains, fruits, and vegetables, the case for including more fiber in your diet is compelling.

A diet heavy in fiber may lower blood cholesterol levels, promote regularity, and prevent gastrointestinal diseases including diverticulitis. Whole-grain foods retain their original fiber, the nutrient-rich bran and germ, and the starchy endosperm in contrast to their processed counterparts, such white rice or white bread.

Although it may sound scholarly, this has a significant impact on nutrition. Most of the nutritious value of whole grains is lost during the refining process that creates refined grains. People mistakenly think that the regulations requiring enriched white flour make up for the numerous beneficial elements lost during processing. Although a few artificial vitamins and minerals are added to our white flour, this does not even come close to making up for all the nutrients that have been lost.

For instance, whole wheat includes selenium, zinc, copper, manganese, phosphorus, sodium, calcium, iron, and magnesium. It also contains vitamin B6, folate, vitamin E, pantothenic acid, vitamin B6, thiamin, and riboflavin.

All carbs are converted by the body into glucose. However, processed grains are broken down considerably more quickly than whole grains. Processed carbohydrates quickly break down, which frequently results in large swings in blood sugar that can lead to cravings for food, the production of stress hormones, and the formation of arterial plaques.

Brown rice, barley, millet, oats, buckwheat, rye, and whole wheat are examples of basic whole grains. In health food stores, you might also want to try some traditional Native American grains like quinoa ("keen-wa") or amaranth. On the internet, it's simple to find delicious whole-grain dishes. But since whole grains typically take longer to cook than refined grains, enjoying these incredibly healthy meals may need some patience.

CHAPTER 6:

Add Lycopene

Supplements containing lycopene are made from carotenoid compounds, which appear naturally as orange, yellow, and red pigments in several plants. Tomatoes, carrots, sweet potatoes, and corn are a few of these. According to a study, lycopene is one of three prevalent carotenoids, the other two being alpha- and beta-carotene. Learn how to profit from lycopene supplements by reading on.

How To Use It

Confront and avert cancer. Lycopene works to prevent the growth of cancers.

Carotenoids-coated living cancer cells inhibit the development of malignancies. They promote the development of healthy cells, and it is advised to eat a variety of them because carotenoids work best in groups.

Additionally, carotenoids prevent LDL cholesterol from creating plaque. Carotenoids avoid arterial blood vessel hardening by delaying the oxidation or hardening of fat. Carotenoids' antioxidant properties enhance the immune system's capacity to combat sickness and infection.

Studies have shown that a diet rich in carotene increases the generation of mononuclear cells, which are essential for the physical function of the immune system. After including tomatoes in their diets, participants in studies on carotenoids increased the synthesis of interleukins, a byproduct of white blood cells that are important to the immune system.

The macular tissue of the eye contains the carotenoids lutein and zeaxanthin. A yellow spot close to the retina's center serves as evidence of their presence. They shield the retina from damaging free radicals and the sun's harmful UV radiation. We must eat meals high in these pigments to prevent macular degeneration as we age and these things start to decline as well.

The active pigment in tomatoes ,Papaya, Pink Grapefruit and Watermelon, "lycopene", gained attention from the general public many years ago when it was discovered that it could prevent prostate cancer.

It was also found that cooking tomato sauce in oil increased the body's absorption of lycopene, which decreased the prevalence of prostatic adenocarcinoma.

Although lycopene hasn't been directly linked to preventing cervical cancer, the American Cancer Society notes that some researchers have determined that lycopene is an antioxidant that lowers the risk of males developing prostate cancer.

Since lycopene is linked to improving the body's ability to fight infection, it might be helpful in curing persistent HPV infections. While many vegetables are healthier when consumed raw or whole, lycopene is more abundant in tomato sauce and tomato juice. Small tomato juice cans stashed at work or in the car can help reduce the desire for unhealthy snacks while also enhancing cervical cancer prevention.

CHAPTER 7:

Get Better Sleep

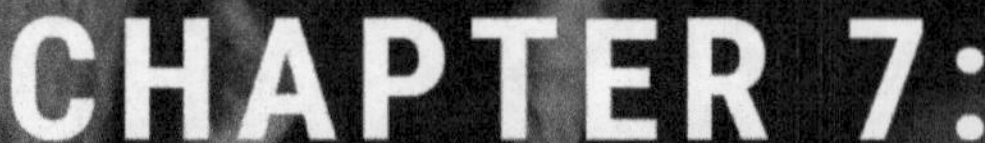

If you've been exercising to reduce your risk of developing cancer, you should be aware that if you aren't getting enough sleep, your extra time spent on the treadmill may not be as beneficial. According to a new study, adult females who are physically active should get at least 7 hours of sleep per night to maximize cancer prevention benefits.

Snooze

Research was carried out in Maryland in 1998 during a period of 9 years, involving adult females aged 18-65. These adult females provided detailed responses to questions In 1998 about their level of activity and typical resting patterns. The following 9 years were covered in terms of cancer data for the group. 604 new cancer cases were reported in the group during this time.

In adult females between the ages of eighteen and sixty-five, those who slept at least seven hours every night and averaged an hour of moderate physical activity each day had a 47 percent lower risk of developing cancer than those who got less sleep on average while maintaining the same level of activity.

The entire cancer prevention benefit comes from being active and getting enough rest, not just sleeping more without physical exertion, says one doctor. "What that indicates to us is that both physical activeness and sleep habits may play a crucial role in reducing cancer risk among younger and middle-aged adult females." You see, getting a good night's sleep has long been linked to health.

In actuality, a lack of sleep has been connected to serious diseases like diabetes, stroke, heart disease, and depression. Another incentive to try to squeeze in those extra hours when you can is the possibility that sleep, especially for active adult females, can help prevent cancer.

You might want to think about your whole lifestyle. Think about various lifestyle choices from a more comprehensive perspective. It is extremely unlikely that one one action may prevent every disease, but by combining many healthy lifestyle practices, you have a far higher chance of maintaining good health.

A balanced diet of natural nutrients, regular exercise, and effective stress management are a few more elements that have a significant impact on your health. If you combine these principles with a restful night's sleep, your body will have a better chance of fending off modern disease.

CHAPTER 8:

Sun Burns Are Bad

Many people are unaware of all the factors involved in preventing skin cancer, sunburn, and premature skin aging. It involves more than just using sunscreen and avoiding the sun's rays during the hottest parts of the day.

Prevent It

The first thing you must do is understand sunrays. UV rays are the sun's rays that cause skin cancer, sunburns, and premature wrinkling of the skin. Further analysis of ultraviolet photons into UVA and UVB rays is possible.

The sunburn-causing UVB rays are to blame. It is summertime and closer to the equator when these rays are strongest since they are closer to the sun. No matter where you are, UVA rays have the same potency and cause premature wrinkling of the skin.

Sunburn can be avoided by using sunscreen with an SPF of 15 or higher to block the UVB rays of the sun. By staying out of the sun's most piercing rays throughout the summer, before 10:00 am, and after 4:00 pm, as well as by staying away from it at the equator and at high altitudes, you can prevent sunburn.

There is more to the equation for preventing skin cancer and premature wrinkles, though. You require broad-spectrum sunscreen or sunscreen that blocks UVA and UVB rays. One brand that offers such comprehensive sun protection is Helioplex.

Where are you going, you might ask? You'll need more sunburn protection if you're traveling to places like the Sunshine State, the Caribbean, or South America than, say, Boston. Use more extensive measures of protection.

A sunblock with SPF 55 and Helioplex is made by Neutrogena, providing the maximum level of protection. If you're going to be on a mountain, the sun's rays are stronger at higher altitudes. You must use UVA and UVB radiation protection with an SPF of 50 or higher, such as a helioplex product. Many windshields only filter UVB sunburn rays if you're driving in your automobile. All exposed skin, including your hands and neck, must be covered with UVB sunscreen.

If sunlight enters your home through a window, it can still cause damage to your skin. Wearing sunblock that blocks UVA rays will ensure that you avoid developing skin cancer and premature aging while indoors.
UVA photons from the sun cause sun damage in tanning beds. Although using a commercial tanning bed does not result in significant sunburn, it can cause skin cancer and premature aging. Choose a tanning bed lamp that is lower. Put on a bronzing accelerator to hasten the melanin production in your skin. SPF 4 or 8 or other low-level UVA sunscreen should also be worn.

Sunburn maintenance is essential if you already have one. Select an Aloe and Vitamin E containing product for sunburn relief and treatment. Aloe soothes skin and aids in sunburn recovery. Your skin's suppleness is improved by vitamin E. By hydrating the skin, sunburn relief lotion may also mitigate UVA light damage.

Use a sun umbrella to protect yourself from the sun's harmful rays when at the beach or while moving around in the hot sun. Freckles could be a sign of skin damage and excessive sun exposure. Particularly if they appear in a cluster on a brand-new area of skin, you shouldn't simply disregard them as normal.

Always keep an eye out for developing moles or freckles since they could be symptoms of skin cancer. Consult a doctor if you think you may be experiencing a skin cancer symptom. Not every piece of clothing shields your skin from the sun's rays.

Cotton offers better protection than lightweight materials.

CHAPTER 9:

A Few Less Drinks

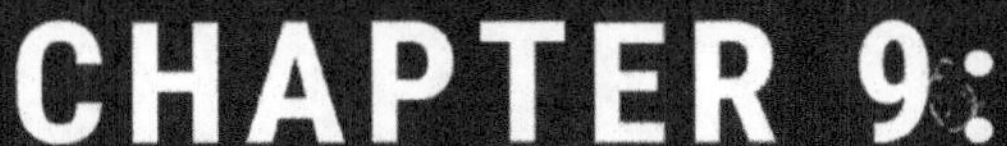

Alcohol intake is regularly linked to an increased risk of cancer, according to a large body of evidence.

Observe The Alcohol

Alcohol consumption increases the risk of liver cancer, female breast cancer, esophageal cancer, intestinal cancer (colon and rectum), and mouth and throat cancer (larynx and pharynx).

The danger of developing cancer is not merely increased by heavy drinking; even small doses of alcohol raise the risk. However, the more alcohol you consume, the greater the risk.

There is no evidence that drinking alcohol helps protect you from any type of cancer, despite some evidence that frequent, little doses of alcohol (like red wine) may lower heart disease in older persons.

All alcoholic beverages, including beer, wine, and spirits, carry the same cancer risk.

What volume should I drink?

You should limit your alcohol intake or, better yet, refrain from it entirely to reduce your risk of developing cancer.
We advise people who do consume alcohol to limit their intake to no more than two standard drinks each day.
We also advise people who drink to avoid binge drinking, which is when they drink heavily for an extended period of time, and to have at least one or two alcohol-free days each week.

Ways To Cut Back On Drinking

- If you do decide to drink, replace alcoholic beverages with non-alcoholic ones like sparkling or plain water (soda with lime and bitters is a fantastic substitute for alcohol).

- Be sure to eat something when drinking alcohol. Consider a glass of wine or beer as something to be consumed alongside food rather than on its own.
- Try a shandy (beer and lemonade) or white wine and mineral water as examples of cut alcoholic beverages.

- Select a wine or beer that is low in alcohol (or alcohol-free).

- Drink water to slake your thirst, and take alcoholic beverages carefully.

- When you go out, offer to be the designated driver to reduce your consumption, but make sure you stay under the legal limit.

CHAPTER 10:

Drop Those Extra Pounds

A BMI of 30 or higher is considered obese and is associated with an increased risk of colorectal cancer. Reducing your BMI lowers your risk of developing colon or rectum cancer by lowering your weight-to-height ratio. The only thing left is weight since you cannot change your height.

Lose Weight

In all other respects, obese men appear to have a higher risk of colon cancer than obese women.

Similar to how specific body shapes tend to affect risk more than others, According to studies, having an apple-shaped waist increases colon cancer risk more than having thighs or hips that are also overweight (a pear shape).

Why does losing weight matter to you?

Many obese people have attempted to lose weight in the past or present. It may therefore appear illogical to say, "Hey, you should really consider slimming down."

Sorry, but all I'll be able to do is increase the pressure.

For adult females and adult men combined, colorectal cancer is the second-leading cause of cancer deaths in the United States.

In actuality, colon cancer claims more lives annually than breast cancer and acquired immune deficiency syndrome. You have good reasons to care about preventing colon cancer if you love yourself and the people who care about you.

What should you do?

Check to discover if you are considered obese (by the CDC), which puts you at a higher risk for colon cancer.

Calculate your BMI to do this. You should try to lose weight (or keep trying) if it's thirty or higher.

I would if I had a quick and straightforward way to help you lose weight. I would also be well off. Unfortunately, I am unaware of any effective short-term solutions for weight loss. But I do have some hints. You must eat sensibly and often exercise if you want to achieve and maintain a healthy weight.

Losing weight is not an easy process. It's frequently frustrating and even depressing.

However, it is not necessary to be that way. You'll lose weight by adopting a healthier diet and more active lifestyle. You will lose weight, though the process may be more arduous than you would like. And once you do, you'll feel better and have reduced your chance of several diseases, including colon cancer.

CHAPTER 11:

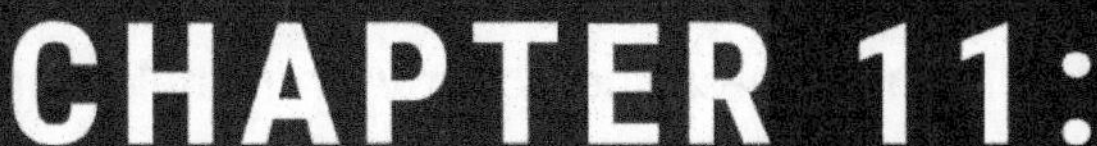

The only condition that kills more people in the United States than cancer is heart disease. More than 500,000 people per year lose their lives to cancer. If more people underwent cancer screenings, many cancer deaths might possibly be prevented.

Screening

Detecting malignancies and pre-cancers early on may lower disease and mortality by screening for colorectal, breast, and cervical cancers. However, many individuals do not get the recommended routine screenings that could save their lives.

Nearly 20% of all cancer deaths in the United States occurred in 2001 as a result of colorectal, breast, and cervical malignancies, according to the CDC's National Center for Health Statistics.

Early detection could significantly reduce the yearly billions spent on cancer treatment. Cancer screening not only saves lives by detecting breast, cervical, and colorectal cancers early, but it also serves as the first step in preventing many cases of colorectal and cervical cancer from ever developing:

• Regular screening could cut the number of people who pass away from colorectal cancer by at least 60%.

• Mammograms performed every 1-2 years on adult females 40 years of age and older may reduce death rates by 20%-25% over ten years.

• Precancerous lesions may be found by Pap tests, allowing for their treatment before cervical cancer spreads. Researchers in numerous nations found that cervical cancer death rates decreased by 20%–60% once screening programs were implemented.

A growing number of American adults are getting examined for cancer every year, and as a result, many are still living and healthy today.

Regular colorectal cancer screening, which should begin at age 50, reduces the incidence and death of the disease, according to sound scientific data. By finding precancerous polyps, colorectal cancer screening can stop cancer from progressing. Similar to lung cancer, colorectal cancer may be found by screening at an early stage when therapy may be most successful.

Deaths from colorectal cancer could be reduced by as much as 60% with routine screening.

Adult females without insurance or with inadequate insurance suffer disproportionately more deaths from breast and cervical cancer.

Women without a regular source of healthcare, adult women without health insurance, and adult women who came to America within the last ten years underutilize mammography and Pap tests.

Conclusion

Many people are affected by cancer. Researchers have identified a large number of chemicals that cause cancer. Making a few key lifestyle changes, like exercising, eating well, avoiding sun exposure, and quitting smoking, can help prevent the majority of cancers.

It's not as simple as taking a pill or receiving a shot to prevent cancer, the top cause of death in the world. However, the World Health Organization (WHO) reports that more than 30% of all.

Deaths from cancer can be avoided. The major problem today is tobacco use.

A deciding aspect of cancer risk. You can include all of them.

using these methods to fight cancer or prevent it and lengthen your life